Can five ancient Tibetan rites really make you look and feel years younger? Here's what readers are saying:

[By the time he reached retirement age, Dr. Joilette was "an overweight, gray-haired wreck, old before my time." He was stooped over and unable to turn his head because of an old neck injury. Since beginning the Five Rites, he reports:] "I have lost twenty pounds, have more energy, and feel more alert. My hair is brown-black and thicker, with only a few streaks of gray at the temples. I have a full range of movement at my neck, without pain, and stand erect. I walk with a light, springy gait. My sexual desires and my abilities have all returned to normal. I cannot explain this medically or scientifically, yet I know that what has happened to me is absolutely true. People who have not seen me for years are astounded. . . ."

—*Russell Joilette, M.D.,*
Hartford, KY

"My muscular strength has improved, my shoulders are straighter, and my abdominal muscles are firmer. After six months, the gray hair at the back of my head began to turn back to its original dark brown. I've gotten my son, who is in medical school, to start doing the Five Rites too."

—*Robert Cope, M.D.,*
Scottsdale, AZ

"In the beginning I was skeptical, but within three months I could see muscles appearing on my formerly flabby body, and my weight went down from 175 to 160, where it has stayed. My wife was underweight, and she gained 8 pounds and feels excellent."

—*B. S. Mell, M.D., Jackson, LA*

"I recommended your book to several patients who later came back with glowing reports. So I began doing the Five Rites myself three weeks ago. After about nine days, I felt a great increase in strength and endurance. I was able to climb stairs with heavy packages without any strain. A nutritionist I recently met told me he performed the Five Rites for four months and became much stronger, even though he was athletic for years and lifted weights regularly. His friends told him he had become younger looking."

—*Dr. Stanley Bass, D.C., Ph.C.,*
Brooklyn, NY

"After one week, I noticed a remarkable change in my health and appearance. Now I look ten years younger and almost never experience aches and pains in spite of a rigorous physical regimen. I recommended the book to my clients, and it has cured them of arthritis, joint problems, chronic pain, weight problems, and I believe a host of emotional and mental problems."

—*Jerry Larkin, Albany, CA*

"Before I read your book, I was only nineteen years old, but felt forty-three. After just a few weeks, I noticed a big difference. I had more energy, lost weight, and got more done. I felt alive. I didn't feel like a forty-three-year-old or a nineteen-year-old either. I felt like a hyperactive ten-year-old. I only needed about five hours of sleep a night instead of the previous ten."

—*Rob Hadley, Kings Mountain, NC*

LOOK YOUNGER

"I have *honestly never felt better in my life!* (I am fifty-six years old.) I have lost weight. I am *strong & energetic & I look and feel fifteen years younger!!!* Not a week goes by that somebody doesn't remark how amazingly young I look. Most say I don't look a day over forty. My children in their mid-thirties are amazed at my energy and youthful looks, so now they are doing the Five Rites."

—*Esther Black, Salinas, CA*

"I not only feel younger, but am told by people who know my age (seventy-three) that I look twenty years younger. My doctor, who is fifty-eight, complained that although he jogs fifteen to twenty miles per week, I look younger than he does. I recommend this book to anyone who wants to halt the aging process."

—*Jack Smithson, Grass Valley, CA*

"Recently a friend of mine began to look much younger, and his full gray beard began to turn a lovely shade of brown. Upon questioning, he told me about the fountain of youth book. Since I started doing the Five Rites, here's what's happened to me: My insomnia and eczema have disappeared completely. My hot flashes said good-bye (I'm fifty-three). After twenty-five years of bifocals, I no longer need glasses. And my eyes have turned a lovely shade of blue, like twenty-five years ago. I feel like I'm sixteen again, but I'm going to miss my lovely silver hair. It's the only thing I liked about being older."

—*Ida Schultz, Salt Lake City, UT*

HAIR TURNS DARK

"The Five Rites seemed like a good exercise program, but frankly, I didn't believe all the wild claims. I am now midway into my fourth week, and for the past eight or so days have noticed my 'pretty' silver-gray hair turning black! I know this sounds crazy, but it's happening right before my eyes. This is weird, but I'm sold on your program."

—*L. C. Nolte, Pasadena, TX*

"My white hair is going back to light brown. *No white hair left.* Don't know the answer to that one."

—*Ellie Stevens, Okanogan, WA*

"When I began the rites, my beard & mustache were gray and my skin so pale, I looked like the ghost of my grandfather. Now my body has a good tone & complexion, and my beard and mustache have gradually changed color until they are nearly black. Also, I can read fine print, something I could never do before."

—*Charles Hamilton, Thousand Oaks, CA*

"For a while, my hair was thinning and coming out. Now it's growing in again and becoming thicker."

—*Henry V., Hawthorn, NJ*

BETTER MEMORY

"At age eighty-three I had lost all interest in life. I was thinking of putting myself in a home, and I didn't think I would live much longer. Then I discovered your book about the Five Rites. I have been doing them only a short time, but already my memory has improved 50 percent, and I feel so much more alive. Everyone tells me I am looking younger all the time. Thanks to the Five Rites, I am a completely different person now, and am continuing to improve. Everyone should read this book."

—*E. B. K. Miller, Buxton, NC*

"My memory was getting so bad, I was ashamed. Now, after using the rites daily for two months, I seem to be getting clarity of mind, and much, much more energy. My friends notice the change too. I am truly thankful that at age sixty-two I am 'youthing' instead of aging."

—*Adeline Neveu, Yakima, WA*

"The physical, emotional, and mental impact is tremendous. I feel better about myself; I'm more alert and generally more pleasant. My mind is quicker and clearer. My posture has improved substantially. I highly recommend this book to anyone of any age."

—*Steven Hunt, Troy, MI*

ARTHRITIS RELIEF

"I had rheumatoid arthritis & was beginning to lose my ability to walk, as my feet and knees had been affected. I also had lots of back pain. I was in such bad shape. Now I can walk several miles & no longer have pain. I believe I would have been in a wheelchair today, if it were not for your book."

—*Janet Matson, Waynesboro, VA*

"Arthritis is very difficult to live with and control. But your book enabled me to stop it and actually reverse the process. It's the best medicine I have ever found. I will treasure it until the end of my time."

—*Ernest Cortez, Corcoran, CA*

"I have arthritis in my left knee. Since I read your book, I've been able to almost completely stop the Naprosyn I was taking. For me, that is a miracle. I had sinus problems for thirty years, but I've been able to stop my sinus medication too. That also is a miracle. I cannot thank you enough for the great health you have given me. I no longer have to take any medications."

—*James Bannon, Lancaster, NY*

"The doctor said I was full of arthritis, and there was nothing I could do about it. Since receiving your book three years ago, I have no more pain and can touch my toes with the palms of my hands. I can now read fine print without my glasses. I have no more sinus problems. And I can outwalk and outwork many friends fifteen to twenty years younger than I am."

—*Lucy Gilbert (age ninety-five), Wellington, KS*

"I have had rheumatoid arthritis for twenty or more years. I was to the point of not being able to get up off the floor without hanging on to something. Also, I had to climb stairs one at a time like a child just learning to walk. Since reading your book, I can climb them again like I should. I can hardly wait to see what happens next."

—*Phyllis Specter, Springfield, OH*

VISION IMPROVEMENT

"In just one week's time, I've noticed a great improvement in my vision, something I regard as remarkable. Another amazing thing—my hands, which looked very, very old, now look better than they have in ten years."

—*Ruth D. Hall, Carson, CA*

"My vision sharpened up, and my friend's eye doctor told her that her eyesight has improved too."

—*Carolyn Carson, San Francisco, CA*

"I have never felt so fit. My body is completely toned—no flab. I'm never tired. I don't need glasses. I recently had an eye test and my sight has never been better. My hair is thick and healthy. My energy and alertness can equal that of any young person half my age."

—*June Seward, Dana Point, CA*

"I was taking medication for angina, stomach ulcers, sinus problems, and was told I was a candidate for prostate cancer. Besides that, I was lame and my eyesight was failing. The symptoms are all but history now. Friends and family cannot understand how I look so much better."

—*Douglas Bly, Spokane, WA*

ENERGY, LASTING POWER

"I used to come home from work feeling absolutely exhausted—even on weekends after getting plenty of sleep. Since doing the rites, I'm always alert and full of energy. This past summer I had more energy than anyone else on my softball team. The change has been absolutely unbelievable."

—*Linda Felder, Silver Spring, MD*

"I used to drag myself half asleep to class in the morning. After I do the rites, though, I feel refreshed and alert, even looking forward to my studies. Also, I'd been working out for quite some time with only mediocre results. Since starting the rites, I've noticed a dramatic improvement in my performance and an increase in how much I can lift. I'm not sure I buy the metaphysical explanation, but I am sure that the Five Rites work— Thank you."

—*Mark Perkins, Lansing, MI*

"I immediately noticed a change in my energy and feeling of well-being. My days flow better, and I have more lasting power on my job.

This is true only when I do the Five Rites."

WEIGHT LOSS

"Before I read your book, I weighed 287 pounds. Now I weigh in at 199. Believe me, IT WORKS!!!"

—Joseph M., Detroit, MI

"Everything this book claims is true. I haven't been sick for one and a half years—not even a cold. Without even trying I went from 179 lbs. to 149. My energy level has risen 100 percent. I don't come home from work dead tired anymore. Although I'm fifty-eight years old, I could pass for early forties. Yours is the best book I have ever purchased."

—John Olson III, Milpitas, CA

"Since I started the rites, I've lost twenty or twenty-five pounds and three inches around my waist, and I've gone from a size forty-four to a size forty! My body really feels at least fifteen years younger, and I continue to grow younger each day."

—Ronald E. Borne, Richardson, TX

"I notice more energy, and I've lost weight (from 190 to 165 pounds). There seems to be a glow around my skin, a healthy color. My wife lost the same weight and inches as I did, and she also lost cellulite around her tummy & legs."

—Eugene Keel, Milledgeville, OH

"I lost twenty-seven pounds and achieved more sexual pleasure."

—Dillon Starr, Clermont, FL

"Within six months the fat and flab began to disappear and muscles began appearing where they had never been before. My only sport is bowling, and at age sixty I became top woman bowler in all three leagues. I will always remember when another bowler said, 'When I come back in my next life, I want a shape like yours.' "

—Grace Carlson, Little River, SC

"The sagging skin on my neck and jaws tightened up. I have more body strength, and facial wrinkles have disappeared. I highly recommend this book to all interested in their health. Those who don't have it don't know what they are missing."

—Michael Roland,
Madison Heights, MI

"I've never found anything before that changes my body shape like this does. I actually have nice legs now, and my breasts are larger. When I followed the instructions in your book, everything seemed to move to the best and proper place."

—Paulette Schmidt, Tucson, AZ

PAIN RELIEF

"Before, I had so many aches and pains: knee pain, shoulder pain, migraines. Now I very seldom have headaches, my knee pain is gone, I never have colds, my sexual ability has been rekindled, and I receive many compliments from people who tell me I look much younger than my age."

—*Casimiro Sanbollo, Honolulu, HI*

"I'm going to be seventy May 1st. Had not your book come along, I would be in a wheelchair living on painkillers. I have deterioration of the bones, and my right knee was getting very bad with the rest of my joints. I'd go up the stairs with my hands on the steps, and I'd come down backwards. Thank God for your book. I now have no pain. When I look in the mirror, my arms are not as flabby. My neck looks better. Most important of all, there's no pain."

—*Mary Reilly, Philadelphia, PA*

"I had a severe lower back condition resulting from a fractured vertebra, nerve damage, and a degenerative disk condition. In addition, I developed a severe pain that ran from the lower back area up the spine to the base of the skull. And frequently I experienced spinal tremors. The first time I did Rite Number Two, as I raised my legs, I felt and heard a snap, a pop, and a crunch in the lower back area. THE PAIN STOPPED. RELIEF WAS IMMEDIATE, AND THE PAIN HAS NOT RETURNED!"

—*Howard F. Stevens, Jr.,*
Bangor, ME

"My sciatic nerve was pinched. It was very painful, and I could only walk a short distance. My doctor said I might have to have surgery and would be confined to a wheelchair for the rest of my life. Then I read your book, began the Five Rites, and I haven't had any pain since."

—*Bernetta Grant, Somerset, PA*

"Several years ago, I fell and injured my back. I was under care of my family doctor, an orthopedic doctor, and a pain specialist. I tried physical therapy, acupuncture, and chiropractic treatments. None helped. Then one day I discovered your book. Three months later, I was my old self again. My friends tell me I'm going backwards. Instead of getting older, I'm getting younger."

—*Lois Masada, San Diego, CA*

"I had a sciatic condition, and for ten years I never went more than four days without some pain or discomfort. On three occasions, the pain was so severe I was incapacitated. Then four weeks ago I started the rites, and I haven't had a twinge or hint of discomfort since. Thank you for introducing me to my own fountain of youth."

—*Fawn Witte, Reno, NV*

"I have a narrowing of the spinal column which causes great pain. Since using your book, I am almost *pain-free*. Also, my kidneys and bladder work more normally. My sinus problem has improved 100 percent. I feel younger, more limber, and just all-around better than I did before."

—*June Tower, Clinton, MD*

"It took a couple of months for me to begin noticing that the lower back pain I had suffered with for fifteen to twenty years had just about disappeared completely. For the last month or two, I think I've actually been getting more hair, thicker hair. I am extremely pleased with my results."

—*Carl Albend, Pine Bluff, AR*

"After the first week, I realized my lower back pain was disappearing. Now, thirteen months later, my knee has recovered about 95 percent, and my lower back pain never bothers me. I had more or less concluded my knee was crippled for life, so now I am a believer."

—*Jeff Perry, Wanblee, SD*

FEEL GREAT

"After two days, I could actually see results. As time goes by, I am seeing further startling improvement. I have purchased a lot of health books, and although they are good ones, nothing has helped me so much in such a short time as your book."

—*Ruth S., Kansas City, MO*

"This is one of the best books I know about at this time. I wish all the good people in the world knew about it."

—*Nina Stewart, Gloucester, MA*

"Thank you for publishing this wonderful book. Once I started to read it, I couldn't put it down. . . . P.S., I'm seventy-seven and have been looking for a book like this all my life!"

—*Evelyn Sugden, Allentown, PA*

ANCIENT SECRET

of the

FOUNTAIN

of

YOUTH

BOOK 1

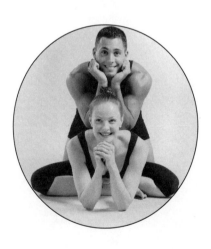

ANCIENT SECRET

of the

FOUNTAIN

of

YOUTH

B O O K 1

Peter Kelder

HARBOR PRESS

Gig Harbor, Washington

PUBLISHED BY HARBOR PRESS, INC.
P.O. Box 1656
Gig Harbor, WA 98335

Book design by Lynn Amft

Library of Congress Cataloging-in-Publication Data
Kelder, Peter.
Ancient secret of the fountain of youth, book 1 / Peter Kelder. —1st ed.
p.   cm.
Originally published: New, rev. ed. Gig Harbour, Wash. : Harbor Press, c1985.
"Book 1."
1. Exercise.   2. Longevity.   3. Rejuvenation.   4. Medicine, Tibetan.   I. Title.
RA781.K36   1998
613.7—dc21   97-34642
                                                                        CIP

ISBN 0-936197-30-7

F O R E W O R D

All wisdom is ancient, and in reality is not a secret. When you think you have discovered something new and previously unknown, it has probably existed for centuries. You didn't know about it, simply because you didn't make the effort to seek it out.

And after all, why should you? Why look to the wisdom of ancient masters if modern science and technology can provide for all your needs and wants? I find that most people think this way until a life-threatening illness occurs. Then they are forced to confront their own mortality, and a different perspective takes hold. As they realize that science and technology offer no solution to the crisis they face, their values and priorities begin to change. They awaken to life. They start to seek out wisdom that will help them engage in life fully and meaningfully. They discover the joy of living.

After years as a practicing physician, I discovered that there are three specific personality traits in people who face life-threatening illness, yet manage to survive longer than expected. They have a fighting spirit, a willingness to learn and change, and spiritual resourcefulness.

Then I recently read the words of a mahatma who said that a healthy individual displays three qualities: action, wisdom, and devotion. In other words, he had written the same thing that had taken me years to discover on my own. If I had sought out his words long ago, I could have used their wisdom to help more people, and I could have saved myself a good deal of time and energy.

In the same manner, this book can save you time and energy. It contains very practical information and a great deal of wisdom which you can use to start the process of *youthing*. And it can help you achieve a healthier and more fulfilling life. As you begin to read its pages and put its wisdom into practice, please keep in mind these few words of advice:

First, as you follow the instructions in this book, be kind to yourself. If you're too demanding, you'll only be setting yourself up for failure. Instead, proceed at your own pace and in your own style. Take delight in your progress, even at times when progress is slow. Remember, youthing is a process, and it can work only so long as you enjoy it.

Next, see yourself as the person you want to be. Studies have shown that body chemistry is altered by the role an actor plays. The truth is, we are all actors on life's stage, and all our lives are shaped by the parts we choose to play. To recast yourself in a different role, change the way you see yourself, and the world will change its perception of you.

And just as actors and athletes rehearse and practice, so must you. Let this book be your coach. Use it not to avoid death, but to enhance the quality of your life. Use it to find greater joy in living. Then be happily surprised by how long you live. Longevity is not the goal; it is the by-product of a healthy life that is lived joyfully.

Finally, never forget that the source of the fountain of youth is *you*. You are in charge. You have the power to activate the life and death mechanisms in your own body. I say this not to blame you, but to empower you.

Don't wait until you are near death before you awaken to life. Begin now to live life fully, and set the youthing process in motion.

Peace,

Bernie S. Siegel, M.D.

ABOUT THE AUTHOR

Peter Kelder was raised by adoptive parents in the midwestern United States, and while still in his teens he left home to embark on adventures that took him around the world to many distant and exotic lands. He became an educated, polished, and articulate man, conversant in many languages, and throughout his life he maintained a love of books, libraries, words, and poetry.

Kelder asserts that Colonel Bradford—the pseudonym for his book's main character—was a real individual who did travel to Tibet and whom he did meet in the 1930s in southern California where his book was written.

However, Kelder is an intensely private man who does not wish to reveal more to the public than these brief details. He feels that his book speaks for itself and that issues concerning himself and Colonel Bradford can serve only to detract from the validity of the simple, straightforward message which is his offering to the world.

While he does not reveal when he was born, Mr. Kelder is very much alive, well, and productive today, nearly sixty years after his book was first published.

PART ONE

*Every man desires to live long,
but no man would be old.*

—Jonathan Swift

One afternoon some years ago, I was sitting in the park reading the afternoon paper when an elderly gentleman walked up and seated himself alongside me. Appearing to be in his late sixties, he was gray and balding, his shoulders drooped, and he leaned on a cane as he walked. Little did I know that from that moment forward, the whole course of my life would change.

It wasn't long before the two of us were engaged in a fascinating conversation. It turned out that the old man was a retired British Army officer who had also served in the diplomatic corps for the Crown. As a result, he had traveled at one time or another to virtually every corner of the globe. And Colonel Bradford, as I shall call him—though it is not his real name—held me spellbound with highly entertaining stories of his adventures. When we parted, we agreed to meet again, and before long, a close friendship had developed between us. Frequently, we got together at his place or mine for discussions and conversations that lasted late into the night.

On one of these occasions, it became clear to me that there was something of importance that Colonel Bradford wanted to talk about, but for some reason he was reluctant to do so. I attempted to tactfully put him at ease, assuring him that if he wanted to tell me what was on his mind, I would keep it in strict confidence. Slowly at first, and then with increasing trust, he began to talk.

While stationed in India some years ago, Colonel Bradford had from time to time come in contact with wandering natives from remote regions of the interior, and he had heard many fascinating stories of their life and customs. One strange tale that particularly caught his interest was repeated quite a number of times, and always by the natives of a particular district. Those from other districts seemed never to have heard of it.

It concerned a group of lamas, or Tibetan clerics, who, according to the story, had discovered the secret of eternal youth. For thousands of years, this extraordinary knowledge had been handed down by members of this particular sect. And though they made no effort to conceal anything, the lamas were completely cut off from the outside world by vast, uninhabited mountain ranges. Their knowledge remained a secret known only to themselves.

This monastery and its fountain of youth had become something of a legend to the natives who spoke of it. They told stories of old men who mysteriously regained health, strength, and vigor after finding and entering the monastery. But no one seemed to know the exact location of this strange and marvelous place.

Like so many other men, Colonel Bradford had become old at the age of forty, and since then had not been growing any younger. The more he heard of this miraculous fountain of youth, the more he became convinced that such a place actually existed. He began to gather information on directions, the character of the country, the climate, and other data that might help him locate the spot. And once his investigation had begun, the Colonel became increasingly obsessed with a desire to find this fountain of youth.

The desire, he told me, had become so irresistible, he had decided to return to India and search in earnest for this retreat and its secret of lasting youth. And Colonel Bradford asked me if I would join him in the effort.

Normally, I would be the first to be skeptical of such

an unlikely story. But the Colonel was completely sincere. And the more he told me of this fountain of youth, the more I became convinced that it could be true. For a while, I was tempted to join the Colonel's search. But as I began to take practical matters into consideration, I finally sided with reason and decided against it.

As soon as Colonel Bradford had left, I began to doubt whether I had made the right decision. To reassure myself, I reasoned that perhaps it's folly to want to conquer aging. Perhaps we should all simply resign ourselves to growing old gracefully and not ask more from life than others expect.

Yet in the back of my mind the haunting possibility remained: a fountain of youth. What a thrilling idea! For his sake, I hoped that the Colonel might find it.

Years passed, and in the press of everyday affairs Colonel Bradford and his Shangri-La grew dim in my memory. Then, one evening on returning to my apartment, I found a letter in the Colonel's own handwriting. I quickly opened it and read a message that appeared to have been written in joyous anticipation. The Colonel said that in spite of frustrating delays and setbacks, he believed that he was actually on the verge of finding the fountain of youth. He gave no return address, but I was relieved to at least know that the Colonel was still alive.

Many more months passed before I heard from him again. When a second letter finally arrived, my hands almost trembled as I opened it. For a moment I couldn't believe its contents. The news was better than I could possibly have hoped. Not only had the Colonel found the fountain of youth, he was bringing it back to the States with him and would arrive sometime within the next two months.

Four years had elapsed since I had last seen my old friend, and I began to wonder how he might have changed in that period of time. Had this fountain of youth enabled him to stop the clock on advancing age? Would he look as he did when I last saw him, or would he appear to be only one year older instead of four?

Eventually the opportunity to answer these questions arrived. While I was at home alone one evening, the house phone rang unexpectedly. When I answered, the doorman announced, "Colonel Bradford is here to see you." A rush of excitement came over me as I responded, "Send him right up." Shortly, the bell rang and I threw open the door. But to my disappointment I saw before me not Colonel Bradford, but another much younger man.

Noting my surprise, the stranger said, "Weren't you expecting me?" And then in a friendly voice he added, "I thought I would be receiving a more enthusiastic welcome. Look closely at my face. Do I need to introduce myself?"

Confusion turned to bewilderment and then amazed disbelief as I stared at the figure before me. Slowly, I realized that the features of his face did indeed resemble those of Colonel Bradford. But this man looked as the Colonel might have looked years ago in the prime of his life. Instead of a stooping, sallow old man with a cane, I saw a tall, straight figure. His face was robust, and he had a thick growth of dark hair with scarcely a trace of gray.

"It is indeed I," said the Colonel, "and if you don't ask me inside, I'll think your manners badly lacking."

In joyous relief I embraced the Colonel, and unable to contain my excitement, I ushered him in under a barrage of questions.

"Wait, wait," he protested good-naturedly. "Allow

yourself to catch your breath, and I'll tell you everything that's happened." And this he proceeded to do.

As soon as he arrived in northern India, the Colonel started directly for the Tibetan frontier and the district where the fabled fountain of youth purportedly existed. Fortunately, he knew quite a bit of the native language, and he spent many months establishing contacts and befriending people. Then he spent many months more putting together the pieces of the puzzle. It was a long, slow process, but persistence finally won him the coveted prize. After a long and perilous expedition into unmapped reaches of the towering Himalayas, he finally found the monastery which, according to legend, held the secret of lasting youth and rejuvenation.

I only wish that time and space permitted me to record all of the things that Colonel Bradford experienced after being admitted to the monastery. Perhaps it is better that I do not, for much of it sounds more like fantasy than fact. The interesting practices of the lamas, their culture, and their utter indifference to the outside world are hard for Westerners to grasp and understand.

In the monastery, older men and women were nowhere to be seen. The lamas good-naturedly referred to the Colonel as The Ancient One, for it had been a very long time since they had seen anyone who looked as old as he. To them, he was a most novel sight.

"For the first two weeks after I arrived," said the Colonel, "I was like a fish out of water. I marveled at everything I saw and at times could hardly believe what was before my eyes. Soon my health began to improve. I was able to sleep soundly at night, and every morning I awoke feeling more and more refreshed and energetic. Before long, I found that I needed my cane only when hiking in the mountains.

"One morning about three months after I arrived, I got the biggest surprise of my life. I had entered for the first time a large, well-ordered room in the monastery, one that was used as a kind of library for ancient manuscripts. At one end of the room was a full-length mirror. For the past two years I had traveled in the wilderness, and in all that time I had not seen my reflection in a mirror. So with some curiosity I stepped before the glass.

"I stared at the image before me with disbelief. My physical appearance had changed so dramatically that I looked fully fifteen years younger than my age. For so many years I had dared to hope that the fountain of youth might truly exist. Now, before my very eyes was physical proof of its reality.

"Words cannot describe the joy and elation which I felt. In the weeks and months ahead, my appearance continued to improve, and the change became increasingly apparent to all who knew me. Before long my honorary title, The Ancient One, was heard no more."

At this point, the Colonel was interrupted by a knock at the door. I opened it to admit a couple who, though they were good friends of mine, had picked an inopportune moment to visit. Concealing my disappointment as best I could, I introduced them to the Colonel, and we all chatted together for a while. Then the Colonel rose and said, "I am sorry that I must leave so early, but I have another commitment this evening. I hope I shall see all of you again soon." But at the door he turned to me and said softly, "Could you have lunch with me tomorrow? I promise, if you do, you'll hear all about the fountain of youth."

We agreed to a time and place, and the Colonel departed. As I returned to my friends, one of them remarked, "He certainly is a fascinating man, but he looks awfully young to be retired from army service."

"How old do you think he is?" I asked.

"Well, he doesn't look forty," answered my guest,

"but from the conversation I would gather he's at least that old."

"Yes, at least," I said evasively. And then I steered the conversation to another topic. I wasn't about to repeat the Colonel's incredible story, at least not until he had fully explained everything.

The next day, after having lunch together, the Colonel and I went up to his room in a nearby hotel. And there at last he told me full details of the fountain of youth.

"The first important thing I was taught after entering the monastery," said the Colonel, "was this: the body has seven energy centers which in English could be called *vortexes*. The Hindus call them *chakras*. They are powerful energy fields, invisible to the eye, but quite real nonetheless. These seven vortexes govern the seven ductless glands in the body's endocrine system, and the endocrine glands, in turn, regulate all of the body's functions, including the process of aging.

"The first vortex (called the *root chakra)* is located at the base of the spine. The second vortex (the *sacral chakra)* is located in the area of the lower abdomen below the navel. The third vortex (the *solar plexus chakra*) is located above the navel and below the chest. The fourth vortex (the *heart chakra*) is located in the center of the chest. The fifth vortex (the *throat chakra*) is located in the throat area. The sixth vortex (the *brow chakra*) is located at the center of the forehead, between the eyebrows. And the seventh, highest vortex (the *crown chakra*) is located at the crown of the head.

"In a healthy body, each of these vortexes revolves at great speed, permitting vital life energy, also called *prana* or *etheric energy,* to flow upward through the endocrine system. But if one or more of these vortexes begins to slow down, the flow of vital energy is inhibited or blocked, and—well, that's just another name for aging and ill health.

"These spinning vortexes extend outward from the flesh in a healthy individual, but in the old, weak, and sickly they hardly reach the surface. The quickest way to regain youth, health, and vitality is to start these energy centers spinning normally again. There are five simple exercises that will accomplish this. Any one of them alone is helpful, but all five are required to get best results. These five exercises are not really exercises at all. The lamas call them *rites,* so that is how I shall refer to them too."

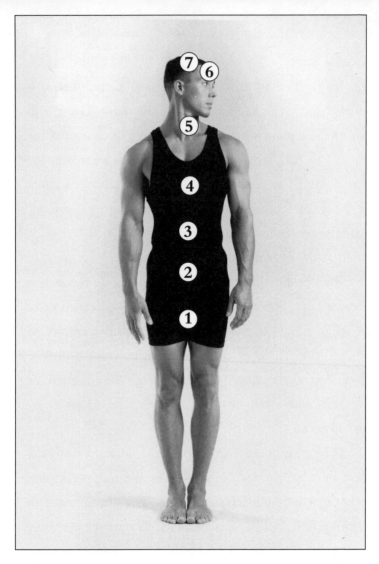

The body's seven energy vortexes govern the seven endocrine glands. They are arrayed in a column in the following manner: (1) the base of the spine; (2) the lower abdomen, below the navel; (3) the upper abdomen, above the navel and below the chest; (4) the center of the chest (5) the throat; (6) the center of the forehead, between the eyebrows; and (7) the crown of the head.

When all seven energy vortexes are revolving at high speed, and at the same rate of speed, the body is in perfect health. When one or more of them slows down, aging and physical deterioration set in.

[Publisher's Caution: Before attempting any of following exercises, read the Appendix on page 101.]

Rite Number One

"The first rite," continued the Colonel, "is a simple one. It is done for the express purpose of speeding up the vortexes. Children do it all the time when they're playing.

"All that you do is stand erect with arms outstretched, horizontal to the floor. Now, without wandering from the spot you are in, slowly spin around until you become slightly dizzy. One thing is important: you must spin from left to right. In other words, if you were to put a clock on the floor faceup, you would turn in the same direction as the clock hands.

"At first, most adults will be able to spin around only about half a dozen times before becoming quite dizzy. As a beginner, don't attempt to do more. And if you feel like sitting or lying down to recover from the dizziness, then by all means do just that. I certainly did at first. To begin with, practice this rite only to the point of slight dizziness. But with time, as you practice all five rites, you will be able to spin more and more times with less dizziness.

"Also, in order to lessen dizziness, you can do what dancers and figure skaters do. Before you begin to spin, focus your vision on a single point straight ahead. As you begin to turn, continue holding your vision on that point as long as possible. Eventually, you will have to let it leave your field of vision, so that your head can spin on around with the rest of your body. As this happens, turn your head around quickly and refocus on your point as soon as you can. This reference point enables you to become less disoriented and dizzy.

"When I was in India, it amazed me to see the Maulawiyah, or as they are more commonly known, the whirling dervishes, almost unceasingly spin around and around in a religious frenzy. After being introduced to Rite Number One, I recalled two things in connection with this practice. First, the whirling dervishes always spun in one direction, from left to right, or clockwise. Second, the older dervishes were virile, strong, and robust. Far more so than most men of their age.

"When I spoke to one of the lamas about this, he informed me that this whirling movement of the dervishes did have a very beneficial effect, but also a devastating one. He explained that their excessive spinning

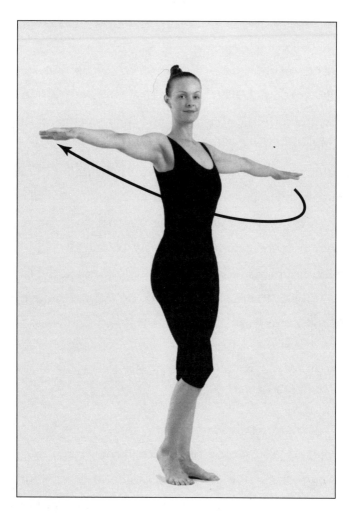

Rite Number One

Standing with your arms outstretched, palms facing downward, spin around in a clockwise direction.

overstimulates some of the vortexes, so that they are finally exhausted. This has the effect of first accelerating the flow of vital life energy, and then blocking it. This building-up and tearing-down action causes the dervishes to experience a kind of psychic rush which they mistake for something spiritual or religious.

"However," continued the Colonel, "the lamas do not carry the whirling to excess. While the whirling dervishes may spin around hundreds of times, the lamas do it only about a dozen times or so, just enough to stimulate the vortexes into action."

Rite Number Two

"Following Rite Number One," continued the Colonel, "is a second rite which further stimulates the seven vortexes. It is even simpler to do. In Rite Number Two, one first lies flat on the floor, faceup. It's best to lie on a thick carpet or some sort of padded surface. The lamas perform the rites on what Westerners might call a prayer rug, about two feet wide and six feet long. It's fairly thick and is made from wool and a kind of vegetable fiber. It is solely for the purpose of insulating the body from the cold floor. Nevertheless, religious significance is attached to everything the lamas do, and hence the name *prayer rug*.

"Once you have stretched out flat on your back, fully extend your arms along your sides and place the palms of your hands against the floor, keeping your fingers close together. Then raise your head off the floor, tucking your chin against your chest. As you do this, lift your legs, knees straight, into a vertical position. If possible, let your legs extend back over your body, toward your head; but do not let your knees bend.

"Then slowly lower both your head and legs, knees straight, to the floor. Allow all of your muscles to relax, and then repeat the rite.

"With each repetition, establish a breathing rhythm: breathe in deeply as you lift your legs and head; breathe out fully as you lower them. Between repetitions, while you're allowing the muscles to relax, continue breathing in the same rhythm. The more deeply you breathe, the better.

"If you are unable to keep your knees perfectly straight, then let them bend as much as necessary. But as you continue to perform the rite, attempt to straighten them as much as you possibly can.

"One of the lamas told me that when he first attempted to practice this simple rite, he was so old, weak,

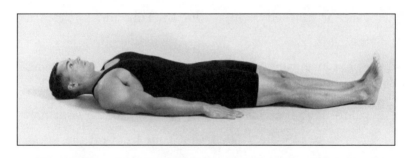

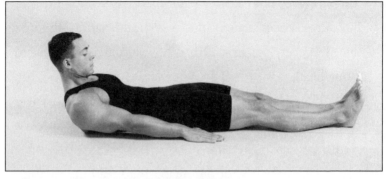

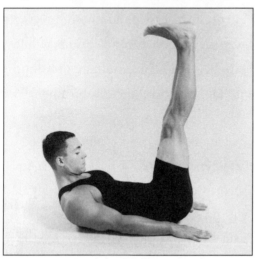

Rite Number Two

1. Lie flat on your back with your arms by your sides.
2. Bring your chin to your chest.
3. Lift your legs to a vertical position, keeping your knees straight.

and decrepit that he couldn't possibly lift his legs into a straight position. So he started by lifting his legs in a bent position, so that his knees were straight up and his feet were hanging down. Little by little, he was able to straighten out his legs until at the end of three months he could raise them straight with perfect ease.

"I marveled at this particular lama," said the Colonel. "When he told me this, he was the perfect picture of health and youth, although I knew he was many years older than I. For the sheer joy of exerting himself, he used to carry a load of vegetables weighing fully a hundred pounds on his back from the garden to the monastery several hundred feet above. He took his time, but never once stopped on the way up. When he arrived, he didn't seem to be in the least exhausted. The first time that I attempted to follow him up the hill, I had to stop at least a dozen times to catch my breath. Later, I was able to climb the hill as easily as he, and without my cane. But that is another story."

Rite Number Three

"The third rite should be practiced immediately after Rite Number Two. It too is a very simple one. All that you need to do is kneel on the floor with both knees bent and the trunk of your body erect. Your hands should be placed at arm's length against your thigh muscles.

"Now, incline your head and neck forward, tucking your chin against your chest. Then gently move your head and neck backward as far as they will go, and at the same time lean backward, arching the spine. As you arch, brace your arms and hands against your thighs for support. After arching, return to the original position and start the rite all over again.

"As with Rite Number Two, you should establish a rhythmic breathing pattern. Breathe in deeply as you arch your spine. Breathe out as you return to an erect position. Deep breathing is most beneficial, so take as much air into your lungs as you possibly can.

"I have seen more than two hundred lamas perform this rite together. In order to turn their attention within, they closed their eyes. In this manner they could eliminate distractions and focus themselves inwardly.

"Thousands of years ago, the lamas discovered that all of the answers to life's imponderable mysteries are found within. They discovered that all of the things which come together to create our lives originate within the individual. Westerners have never been able to understand and comprehend this concept. They think, as I

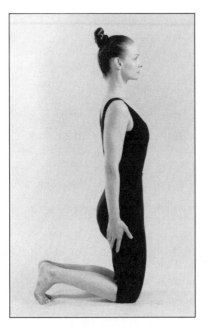

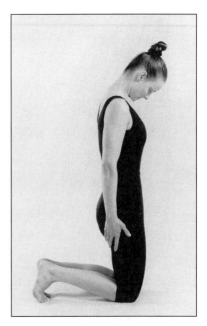

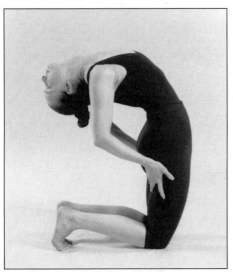

Rite Number Three

1. Kneel on the floor with your body upright. Place your hands against your thighs.
2. Bring your chin to your chest.
3. Arch your spine as you gently move your head backward as far as it will go.

did, that our lives are shaped by the uncontrollable forces of the material world. For example, most Westerners think it is a law of nature that our bodies must grow old and deteriorate. By looking within, the lamas know this to be a self-fulfilling illusion.

"The lamas, especially those at this particular monastery, are performing a great work for the world. It is performed, however, on the astral plane. From this plane they assist humanity around the globe, for it is high above the vibrations of the physical world and is a powerful focal point where much can be accomplished with little loss of effort.

"One day the world will awaken in amazement to see the result of great works performed by these lamas and other unseen forces. The time is fast approaching when a new age will dawn and a new world will be seen. It will be a time when people learn to liberate powerful forces within themselves to overcome war and pestilence, hatred and bitterness.

"We call ourselves civilized, but in truth we are living in the darkest of dark ages. However, we are being prepared for better and more glorious things. Each one of us who strives to raise his or her consciousness to higher levels helps to elevate the consciousness of mankind as a whole. So performing the Five Rites has an impact far beyond the physical benefits which they achieve."

Rite Number Four

"The first time I performed Rite Number Four," said the Colonel, "it seemed very difficult. But after a week, it was as simple to do as any of the others.

"First, sit down on the floor with your legs straight out in front of you and your feet placed apart about the width of your shoulders. With the trunk of your body erect, place the palms of your hands on the floor alongside your buttocks, fingers pointing toward your toes. Then tuck your chin forward against your chest.

"Now let your head sink backward as far as it will go. At the same time, raise your body so that your knees bend while your arms remain straight. The trunk of your body will be in a straight line with your upper legs, horizontal to the floor. And both your arms and lower legs will be straight up and down, perpendicular to the floor. Then tense every muscle in your body. Finally, relax your muscles as you return to the original sitting position and rest before repeating the procedure.

"Again, breathing is important to this rite. Breathe in deeply as you raise your body. Hold in your breath as

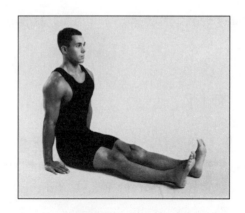

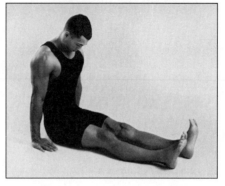

1. Sit on the floor with your legs outstretched, your feet apart, and your hands on the floor.
2. Bring your chin to your chest.

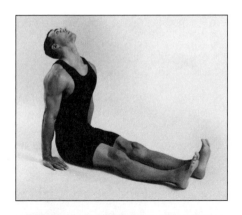

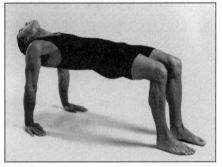

3. Let your head sink back as far as it will go.
4. Keeping your arms straight and your hands and feet in place, bend your knees and raise the trunk of your body to a horizontal position. Tense your muscles, then relax.

you tense your muscles. And breathe out completely as you come down. While you rest between repetitions, continue breathing in the same rhythm.

"After leaving the monastery," continued Colonel Bradford, "I went to a number of larger cities in India, and as an experiment I conducted separate classes in English and Hindustani. I found that the older members of either group felt that unless they could perform this rite perfectly from the very start, no good could come of it. It was extremely difficult to convince them that they were wrong. Finally, I persuaded them to do the best they could just to see what might happen in a month's time. Once I got them to simply do their best in attempting the rites, the results in one month's time were more than gratifying.

"I remember that in one city I had quite a few elderly people in one of my classes. In attempting this particular rite—number four—they could just barely get their bodies off the floor; they couldn't come close to reaching a horizontal position. In the same class there were some much younger persons who had no difficulty performing the rite perfectly the very first day. This so discouraged the older people that I had to separate the two groups. I explained to the older group that when I first attempted this rite, I couldn't perform it any better than they. 'But,' I told them, 'I can now perform fifty repetitions of the rite without feeling the slightest nervous or muscular strain.' And to prove it, I did it right before their eyes. From then on, the older group broke all records for progress.

"The only difference between youth and vigor, and old age and poor health is simply the rate of speed at which the vortexes are spinning. Normalize the rate of speed, and the old person becomes like new again."

Rite Number Five

The Colonel went on, "When you perform the fifth rite, your body will be facedown on the floor. Throughout this rite your hands should be positioned palms-down to the floor, and your feet should be in a flexed position, toes-down to the floor. Both your feet and hands should be spaced apart more or less the width of your shoulders, and your arms and legs should be kept straight.

"Start with your arms straight, perpendicular to the floor, and your spine arched, so that your body is in a sagging position. Now gently move your head backward as far as possible. Then, bending at the hips, bring your body up into an inverted V position. At the same time, bring your chin forward, tucking it against your chest. That's all there is to it. Return to the original position and start the rite all over again.

"By the end of the first week, the average person will find this rite one of the easiest to perform. Once you become proficient at it, let your body drop from the raised position to a point almost, but not quite, touching the floor. Tense your muscles for a moment both at the raised point and at the low point.

"Follow the same deep breathing pattern used in the previous rites. Breathe in deeply as you raise your body. Breathe out fully as you lower it.

"Everywhere I go," continued the Colonel, "people at first call these rites isometric exercises. It's true that the Five Rites are helpful in stretching stiff muscles and joints and improving muscle tone. But that is not their primary purpose. The real benefit of the rites is to normalize the speed of the spinning vortexes. It starts them spinning at a speed which is right for, say, a strong and healthy man or woman twenty-five years of age.

"In such a person," the Colonel explained, "all of the vortexes are spinning at the same rate of speed. On the other hand, if you could see the seven vortexes of the average middle-aged man or woman, you would notice right away that some of them had slowed down

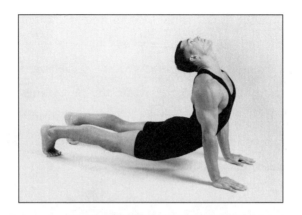

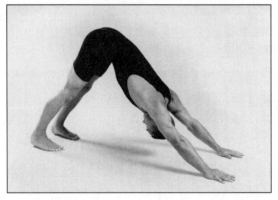

Rite Number Five

1. Support your body in a sagging position with your arms straight, your hands planted on the floor, and your toes curled under. Gently move your head back as far as it will go.
2. Keeping your hands and feet in place, bend at the hips and bring your body into an inverted V position. Bring your chin forward to your chest.

greatly. All of them would be spinning at a different rate of speed, and none of them would be working together in harmony. The slower ones would be causing that part of the body to deteriorate, while the faster ones would be causing nervousness, anxiety, and exhaustion. It is the abnormal condition of the vortexes that produces abnormal health, deterioration, and old age."

As the Colonel was describing the Five Rites, questions were popping into my mind. And now that he was finished, I began to ask a few.

"How many times is each rite performed?" was my first question.

"To start with," replied the Colonel, "I suggest that you practice each rite three times a day for the first week. Then, every week that follows, increase the daily repetitions by two until you are performing each rite twenty-one times a day. In other words, the second week, perform each rite five times; the third week, perform each rite seven times; the fourth week, perform each rite nine times daily; and so on. In ten weeks' time, you'll be doing the full number of twenty-one rites per day.

"If you have difficulty practicing the first rite, the whirling one, as many times as you do the others, then simply do it as many times as you can without getting too dizzy. Eventually you'll be able to whirl around the full twenty-one times.

"I knew a man who performed the rites more than a year before he could spin around that many times. He had no difficulty in performing the other four rites, so he increased the spinning very gradually, until he was doing the full twenty-one. And he got splendid results.

"There are a few people who find it difficult to spin around at all. Usually, if they omit the spinning and perform the other four rites for four to six months, they find that they can then start to handle the spinning too."

"What time of day should the rites be performed?" was my next question to the Colonel.

"They can be performed either in the morning or at night," he answered, "whichever is more convenient. I perform them both morning and night, but I would not advise so much stimulation for the beginner. After you have been practicing the rites for about four months, you might start performing them the full number of times in the morning, and then at night perform just three repetitions of each rite. Gradually increase these as you did before, until you are performing the full twenty-one. But it isn't necessary to perform the rites more than twenty-one times either morning or night. Attempt more only if you are truly motivated to do so."

"Is each of these rites equally important?" I asked next.

"The Five Rites work hand in hand with each other, and all are equally important," said the Colonel. "After performing the rites for a while, if you find that you are not able to do all of them the required number of times, try splitting the rites into two sessions: one in the morning and one in the evening. If you find it impossible to do one of the rites at all, omit it and do the other four. Then, after a period of months, try the one you were having difficulty with again. Results may come a little more slowly this way, but they will come nevertheless.

"Under no circumstances should you ever strain yourself. That would be counterproductive. Simply do as much as you can handle and build up gradually. And never allow yourself to become discouraged. With time and patience there are very few people who cannot eventually perform all five rites twenty-one times a day.

"In attempting to overcome a difficulty with one of the rites, some people become very inventive. An old fellow in India found it impossible to properly perform Rite Number Four even once. He wouldn't be satisfied with just getting his body off the floor. He was determined that his torso should reach a fully horizontal position. So he got a box about ten inches high and padded the top of it. Then he lay down flat upon the box, placing his feet on the floor at one end and his hands on the floor at the other. From this position he was able to raise his torso to a horizontal position quite nicely.

"Now, this gimmick may not have enabled the old gentleman to perform the rite the full twenty-one times. But it did make it possible for him to raise his body as high as much stronger men were able to. And this had a positive psychological effect, which in itself was quite beneficial. I do not particularly recommend his technique, but it could help others who think it's impossible to make progress any other way. If you have an inventive mind, you'll be able to think of other ways and means to help yourself perform any rite that may be particularly difficult for you."

Then I asked the Colonel, "What if one of the rites were left out entirely?"

"These rites are so powerful," he said, "that if one were left out, while the other four were practiced regularly the full number of times, excellent results would still be experienced. Even the first rite alone will do wonders, as the whirling dervishes, whom I spoke of earlier, demonstrate. The older dervishes, who did not spin around so excessively as the younger ones, were strong and virile—a good indication that just one rite can have powerful effects. So if you find that you simply cannot perform all of the rites or that you cannot perform them the full twenty-one times, be assured that you will get good results from whatever you are able to do."

I next asked, "Can the rites be performed in conjunction with other exercise programs, or would the two conflict?"

"By all means," said the Colonel, "if you already have some kind of exercise program, continue it. If you don't, then think about starting one. Any form of exercise—but especially exercise that gives the heart and lungs a good workout—will help the body maintain a youthful equilibrium. In addition, the Five Rites will help to normalize the spinning vortexes, so that the body becomes even more receptive to the benefits of exercise."

"Have you any further suggestions," I asked.

"There are two more things which would help. I've already mentioned deep rhythmic breathing while resting between repetitions of the rites. In addition, between each of the rites, it would be helpful to stand erect with your hands on your hips, breathing deeply and rhythmically several times. As you breathe out, imagine that any tension which may be in your body is draining away, allowing you to feel quite relaxed and at ease. As you breathe in, imagine that you are filling yourself with a sense of well-being and fulfillment.

"The other suggestion is to take either a tepid bath or a cool, but not a cold one after practicing the rites. Going over the body quickly with a wet towel, and then with a dry one is probably even better. One thing I must caution you against: you must never take a shower, tub, or wet towel bath which is cold enough to chill you internally. If you do, you will have undone all of the good you have gained from performing the rites."

I was excited at all the Colonel had told me, but deep down inside there must have been some lingering skepticism. "Is it possible that the fountain of youth is really as simple as what you have described to me?" I asked.

"All that is required," answered the Colonel, "is to practice the Five Rites three times a day to begin with and to gradually increase until you are performing each one twenty-one times a day. That is the wonderfully simple secret that could benefit all the world if it were known.

"Of course," he added, "you must practice the rites every day in order to achieve real benefits. You may skip one day a week, but never more than that. And if you allow a business trip or some other commitment to interrupt this daily routine, your overall progress will suffer.

"Fortunately, most people who begin the Five Rites find it not only easy, but also enjoyable and rewarding to perform them every day, especially when they begin to see the benefits. After all, it takes only twenty minutes or so to do all five. And a physically fit person can perform the rites in ten minutes or less. If you have trouble finding even that much spare time, then just get up a few minutes earlier in the morning or go to bed a little later at night.

"The Five Rites are for the express purpose of restoring health and youthful vitality to the body. Other factors help determine whether you will dramatically transform your physical appearance, as I have done. Two of these are mental attitude and desire.

"You've noticed that some people look old at forty, while others look young at sixty. Mental attitude is what makes the difference. If you are able to see yourself as young, in spite of your age, others will see you that way too. Once I began practicing the rites, I made an effort to erase from my mind the image of myself as a feeble old man. Instead, I fixed in my mind the image of myself when I was in the prime of life. And I put energy in the form of very strong desire behind that image. The result is what you see now.

"For many people this would be a difficult feat because they find it impossible to change the way they see themselves. They believe the body is programmed to sooner or later become old and feeble, and nothing will shake them from that view. In spite of this, once they begin to practice the Five Rites, they will begin to feel younger and more energetic. This will help them to change the way they see themselves. Little by little, they will begin to see themselves as younger. And before long, others will be commenting that they have a younger appearance.

"There is one other extremely important factor for those who want to look dramatically younger. There is an additional rite which I've intentionally been holding back on. But Rite Number Six is a subject which I'll save for a later time."

PART TWO

No man is free who is a slave to the flesh.

—Lucius Annæus Seneca

It had been almost three months since Colonel Bradford's return from Tibet and India, and a great deal had happened in that time. I had immediately begun practicing the Five Rites and was greatly pleased with the excellent results. The Colonel had been away tending to personal matters, so I had been out of contact with him for some time. When he finally phoned me again, I eagerly told him all about my progress, and I assured him that I had already demonstrated to my complete satisfaction how very effective the rites can be.

In fact, I had become so enthusiastic about the rites, I was eager to pass the information on to others who might also benefit. So I asked the Colonel if he would consider leading a class. He agreed that it was a good idea and said that he would do it, but only on three conditions.

The first condition was that the class must contain a cross section of men and women from all walks of life: professionals, blue-collar workers, homemakers, and so on. The second condition was that no member of the class could be under fifty years of age, though they could be a hundred or more if I could find anyone that old willing to participate. The Colonel insisted on this, even though the Five Rites are equally beneficial to younger people. And the third condition was that the class be limited to fifteen members. This came as a considerable disappointment to me because I had envisioned a much larger group. After trying without success to persuade the Colonel to change his mind, I agreed to all three conditions.

Before long, I had managed to assemble a group that met all of the requirements, and right from the beginning the class was a huge success. We met once a week, and as early as the second week, I thought I could see signs of improvement in several of its members. However, the Colonel had asked us not to discuss our progress with one another, and I had no way of knowing whether the others would agree. Then, at the end of the month, my uncertainty was put to rest. We held a kind of testimonial meeting at which all of us were invited to share our results. Everyone present reported at least some improvement. Some had glowing accounts of progress, and a few of these could even be called remarkable. A man nearly seventy-five had made more gains than any of the others.

Weekly meetings of the Himalaya Club, as we named it, continued. When the tenth week finally came, practically all of the members were performing all of the Five Rites twenty-one times a day. All claimed not only to be feeling better, they also believed that they were looking younger, and several even joked that they were no longer telling their real ages.

This reminded me that when we had asked the Colonel his age some weeks back, he had said that he would hold that information until the end of the tenth week. Well, the time had arrived, but as yet the Colonel hadn't put in an appearance. Someone suggested that each of us guess the Colonel's age and write it on a slip of paper. Then, when the truth was announced, we could see who came closest. We agreed to do this, and the slips of paper were being collected as Colonel Bradford walked in.

When we explained what we were up to, Colonel

Bradford said, "Bring them here, so I can see how well you've done. And then I'll tell you what my age really is." In an amused voice, the Colonel read each of the slips aloud. Everyone had guessed him to be in his forties, and most had guessed the early forties.

"Ladies and gentlemen," he said, "thank you for your very generous compliments. And since you've been honest with me, I'll be the same with you. I shall be seventy-three years of age on my next birthday."

At first, everyone stared at him in disbelief. Was it really possible for a seventy-three-year-old man to look nearly half his age? Then, it occurred to them to ask, why had the Colonel achieved results so much more dramatic than their own?

"In the first place," the Colonel explained, "you have been doing this wonderful work for only ten weeks. When you have been at it two years, you will see a much more pronounced change. But there's more to it than just that. I haven't told you all there is to know.

Rite Number Six

"I have given you five rites which are for the purpose of restoring youthful health and vitality. They will

46

also help you regain a younger appearance. But if you really want to completely restore the health and appearance of youth, there is a sixth rite which you must practice. I've said nothing about it up until now because it would have been useless to you without having first obtained good results from the other five."

The Colonel warned them that in order to take advantage of this sixth rite, they would have to accept a very difficult self-restraint. He suggested that they take some time to consider whether they were willing to do this for the rest of their lives. And he invited those who wished to go on with Rite Number Six to return the following week. After thinking it over, only five of the group came back, though the Colonel said this was a better showing than he had experienced with any of his classes in India.

When he told them about this additional rite, the Colonel made it clear that it would lift up the body's reproductive energy. This lifting-up process would cause not only the mind to be renewed, but the entire body as well. But he warned that this would entail a restriction which most people were unwilling to accept. The Colonel continued with this explanation.

"In the average man or woman, part—often a large part—of the vital life force that feeds the seven vortexes is channeled into reproductive energy. So much of it is dissipated in the lower vortexes that it never has a chance to reach the higher ones.

"In order to become a superman or superwoman, this powerful life force must be conserved and turned upward, so that it can be utilized by all of the vortexes, especially the seventh. In other words, it is necessary to become celibate, so that reproductive energy can be rechanneled to a higher use.

"Now turning this vital life force upward is a very simple matter, and yet through the centuries people attempting it have usually failed. In the West, whole religious orders have tried this very thing and failed because they sought to master reproductive energy by suppressing it. There is only one way to master this powerful urge, and that is not by dissipating or suppressing it, but by *transmuting* it, and at the same time lifting it upward. In this way, you have not only discovered the *elixir of life,* as the ancients called it, you have also put it to use, which is something the ancients were seldom able to do.

"Now Rite Number Six is the easiest thing in the world to perform. It should be practiced only when you feel an excess of sexual energy and there is a natural desire for its expression. Fortunately, this rite is so simple that you can do it anywhere, at any time, whenever the urge is felt. Here's all you do:

"Stand straight up and slowly let all of the air out of your lungs. As you do this, bend over and put your hands on your knees. Force out the last trace of air, and then, with your lungs empty, return to a straight-up posture. Place your hands on your hips and press down on them. This will push your shoulders up. As you do this, pull in the abdomen as much as possible and at the same time raise your chest.

"Now hold this position as long as you possibly can. When you are finally forced to take air into your empty lungs, let the air flow in through your nose. When your lungs are full, breathe out through your mouth and relax your arms, letting them hang naturally at your sides. Then, through either your nose or your mouth, breathe in and out deeply several times. This constitutes one complete performance of Rite Number Six. About three repetitions are required for most people to redirect sexual energy and turn its powerful force upward.

"There is only one difference between a person who is healthy and vital and one who is a superman or superwoman. The former channels the vital life force into sexual energy, while the latter turns this force up-

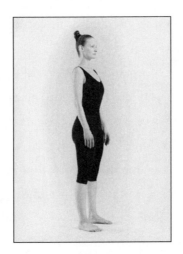

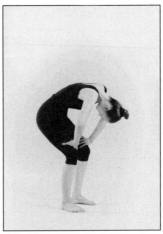

<u>Rite Number Six</u>

1. In a standing position, breathe out fully.
2. Bend over and prop your hands on your knees. Force out the last trace of air.

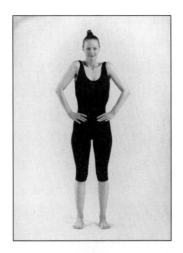

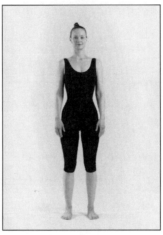

3. Return to a standing position. Place your hands on your hips and press down, forcing your shoulders up. Pull in your abdomen and raise your chest. Hold as long as possible.
4. Breathe in deeply through your nose. Breathe out through your mouth as you relax your arms. Breathe deeply in and out several times.

ward to create balance and harmony through all of the seven vortexes. That's why a superman or superwoman grows younger and younger day by day and moment by moment. They create within themselves the true elixir of life.

"Now you can understand that the fountain of youth was within me all the time. The Five Rites—or six, to be more precise—were merely a key that unlocked the door. When I recall Ponce de León and his futile search for the fountain of youth, I think what a pity it was that he journeyed so far in order to come up empty-handed. He could have achieved his goal without ever leaving home. But like me, he believed that the fountain of youth must be in some distant corner of the world. He never suspected that all the time it was right within himself.

"Please understand that in order to perform Rite Number Six, it is absolutely necessary that an individual have active sexual urge. He or she could not possibly transmute reproductive energy if there were little or nothing to work with. It is absolutely impossible for a person who has lost sexual urge to perform this rite. He or she should not even attempt it because it would only lead to discouragement and more harm than good. Instead, such an individual, regardless of age, should first practice the other five rites, until they regain a normal sexual urge. When this is achieved, he or she may then go into the business of being a superman or superwoman.

"Also, an individual should not attempt Rite Number Six unless he or she is genuinely motivated to do so. If an individual feels incomplete in terms of sexual expression and must struggle to overcome its attraction, then that individual is not truly capable of transmuting reproductive energy and directing it upward. Instead, energy will be misdirected into struggle and inner conflict. The sixth rite is only for those who feel sexually complete and who have a real desire to move on to different goals.

"For the great majority of people, a celibate life is simply not a feasible choice, and they should perform the first five rites only. However, in time the Five Rites may lead to a changing in priorities and a genuine desire to become a superman or superwoman. At that time, the individual should make a firm decision to begin a new way of life. Such an individual must be ready to move forward without wavering or looking back. Those who are capable of this are on their way to becoming true masters, able to use vital life force energy to achieve anything they desire.

"I repeat, let no one think of turning sexual currents upward until they are prepared to leave physical needs behind in exchange for the rewards of true mastership. Then let that individual step forward, and success will crown their every effort."

PART THREE

To lengthen thy life, lessen thy meals.

—Benjamin Franklin

After the tenth week, Colonel Bradford no longer attended each meeting but did keep up his interest in the Himalaya Club. From time to time, he would speak to the group on various helpful subjects, and occasionally members of the group asked advice on something in particular. For example, several of us were especially interested in diet and the tremendously important role that food plays in our lives. There were differing views on the subject, and so we decided to ask Colonel Bradford to describe to us the lamas' diet and their policy concerning foods.

"In the Himalayan monastery where I was a neophyte," said the Colonel when he spoke to us the following week, "there are no problems concerning the right foods, nor in getting sufficient quantities of food. Each of the lamas does his share of work in producing what is needed. All the work is done in the most primitive way. Even the soil is spaded by hand. Of course, the lamas could use oxen and plows if they wished, but they prefer direct contact with the soil. They feel that handling and working the soil adds something to one's existence. I personally found it to be a thoroughly rewarding experience. It contributed to a feeling of oneness with nature.

"Now it is true that the lamas are vegetarian, but not strictly so. They do use eggs, butter, and cheese in quantities sufficient to serve certain functions of the brain, body, and nervous system. However, they do not eat flesh, for the lamas, who are strong and healthy and who practice Rite Number Six, seem to have no need of meat, fish, or fowl.

"Like myself, most of those who joined the ranks of the lamas were men of the world who knew little about proper food and diet. But not long after coming to the monastery, they invariably began to show wonderful signs of physical improvement. And this was due in part at least to their diet there.

"No lama is choosy about what he eats. He can't be because there is little to choose from. A lama's diet consists of good, wholesome food, but as a rule it consists of only one item of food at a meal. That in itself is an important secret of health.

"Different types of food—for example, starches and proteins—require completely different digestive processes in the stomach. So if a starch such as bread is eaten together with a protein such as meat, each one interferes with the digestion of the other. The end result is that neither the bread nor the meat is fully digested; a good part of the food's nutritional value is lost; bloating and physical distress occur; and valuable energy, which could be put to a better use, is depleted in the process. If this state of affairs is permitted to continue over a period of years, your digestive system will begin to decline, your general health will suffer, and your life will be shortened.

"When one eats just one kind of food at a time there can be no clashing of foods in the stomach. Digestion proceeds efficiently with little loss of energy, and the body receives more nourishment from less food.

"Many times in the monastery dining hall, I sat down to the table along with the lamas and ate a meal consisting only of bread. At other times, we ate nothing but fresh vegetables and fruits. At other meals, we ate nothing but cooked vegetables and fruits.

"At first, I was hungry for my usual diet and the

variety of foods which I had been accustomed to. But before long, I could eat and enjoy a meal consisting of nothing but dark bread or just one kind of fruit. Sometimes a meal of just one vegetable would seem like a feast.

"Now, I'm not suggesting that you limit yourself to a diet of just one kind of food per meal or even that you eliminate meats from your diet. But I would recommend that you keep starches, fruits, and vegetables separate from meats, fish, and fowl at your meals. It is all right to make a meal of just meat. In fact, if you wish, you could have several kinds of meat in one meal. And it is all right to eat butter, eggs, and cheese with a meat meal or dark bread and, in moderation, coffee or tea. But you must not end up with anything sweet or starchy—no pies, cakes, or puddings.

"Butter seems to be a neutral. It can be eaten with either a starchy meal or with a protein meal. However, fats in general should be avoided, though not completely eliminated from the diet. The harmful fats are those from animal sources, while the beneficial ones are those contained in seeds, grains, fruits, and vegetables. A small amount of butter is permissible, as is lean meat eaten in limited quantities. But it's best to dispense with pork in any form.

"White sugar, as well as all foods containing white sugar, should be consumed sparingly. Honey and natural sweets can be used instead, and even they should be used in moderation.

"During my stay at the monastery, another interesting and useful thing I learned was the proper use of eggs. The lamas would not eat whole eggs unless they had been performing hard manual labor. Then they might eat one whole medium boiled egg. But they would frequently eat raw egg yolks, discarding the whites. At first, it seemed to me to be a waste of perfectly good food to throw the whites to the chickens. But then I learned that egg whites are utilized only by the muscles and should not be eaten unless the muscles are exercised.

"I had always known that egg yolks are nutritious, but I learned of their true value only after talking with another Westerner at the monastery, a man who had a background in biochemistry. He told me that common hen eggs contain fully half of the elements required by the brain, nerves, and organs of the body. It is true that these elements are needed only in small quantities, but they must be included in the diet if you are to be exceptionally robust and healthy, both mentally and physically.

"There is one more very important thing which I learned from the lamas. They taught me the importance of eating slowly, not for the sake of good table manners, but for the purpose of masticating my food more thoroughly. Mastication is the first important step in breaking down food, so that it can be assimilated by the body. Everything one eats should be digested in the mouth before it is digested in the stomach. If you gulp down food, bypassing this vital step, it is literally dynamite when it reaches the stomach.

"Protein foods such as meat, fish, and fowl require less mastication than complex starches. It is just as well to chew them thoroughly anyway. The more completely food is masticated, the more nourishing it will be. This means that if you thoroughly chew your food, the amount you eat can be reduced, often by one half.

"Many things which I had taken for granted before entering the monastery seemed shocking when I left it two years later. One of the first things I noticed when I arrived in one of the major cities of India was the large amount of food consumed by everyone who could afford to do so. I saw one man eat in just one meal a quantity of food sufficient to feed and completely nourish four hardworking lamas. But of course the lamas would never dream of putting into their stomachs the combinations of food which this man consumed.

"The conglomeration of foods in one meal was another thing that appalled me. Having been in the habit of eating one or two foods at a meal, I was amazed to count twenty-three varieties of food one evening at my host's table. No wonder Westerners have such miserable health. They seem to know little or nothing about the relationship of diet to health and strength.

"The right foods, the right combinations of food, the right amounts of food, and the right method of eating combine to produce wonderful results. If you are overweight, it will help you reduce. And if you are underweight, it will help you gain. There are quite a few other points about food and diet that I would like to go into, but time doesn't permit. Just keep in mind these five things:

1. Never eat starch and meat at the same meal, though if you are strong and healthy, it need not cause you too much concern now.
2. If coffee bothers you, drink it black, using no milk or cream. If it still bothers you, eliminate it from your diet.

3. Chew your food to a liquid and cut down on the amount of food you eat.

4. Eat raw egg yolks* once a day, every day. Take them either just before or after meals—not during the meal.

5. Reduce the variety of foods you eat in one meal to a minimum.

"It's a very simple matter to live simply in our complex world," continued Colonel Bradford. "Just because the world is a complicated place, you don't have to join in the game. Instead, let simplicity guide you in matters of diet and in all things pertaining to mental and physical well-being."

---

* The USDA recommends against the consumption of raw eggs, which can be contaminated with salmonella bacteria and can cause food poisoning.

PART FOUR

A feeble body enfeebles the mind.

—Jean-Jacques Rousseau

Colonel Bradford was addressing the Himalaya Club for the last time before leaving to travel to other parts of the United States and his native England. He had chosen to speak on various things other than the Five Rites which help in the rejuvenation process. And as he stood before the group, he appeared to be sharper, more alert, and more vigorous than ever before. Immediately after his return from India, he had seemed to be the image of perfection. But since then he had continued to improve, and even now he was making new gains.

"First of all," said the Colonel, "I must apologize to the women in our group because much of what I have to say tonight will be directed to the men. Of course, the Five Rites which I have taught you are equally beneficial to men and women. But being a man myself, I would like to speak on a subject of importance to other men.

"I'll begin by talking about the male voice. Do you know that some experts can tell how much sexual vitality a man has just by listening to him speak? We have all heard the shrill, piping voice of a man who is advanced in age. Unfortunately, when an older man's voice begins to take on that pitch, it's a sure sign that physical deterioration is well under way. Let me explain.

"The fifth vortex in the throat area governs the vocal cords, and it also has a direct connection with the second vortex, which governs the body's sexual center. Of course, all of the vortexes have common connections, but these two are, in a manner of speaking, geared together. What affects one affects the other. As a result, when a man's voice is high and shrill, it's an indicator that his sexual vitality is low. And if energy in the second vortex is low, you can bet that it's lacking in the other six as well.

"Now all that's necessary to speed up the second and fifth vortexes, along with all the others, is to practice the Five Rites. But there is another method which you can use to help speed up the process. It's easy to do. All that's required is willpower. You simply need to consciously make the effort to lower your voice. Listen to yourself speak, and if you hear yourself becoming higher or more shrill, adjust your voice to a lower register. Listen to men who have good, firm speaking voices and take note of the sound. Then, whenever you speak, keep your voice down in that masculine pitch as much as possible.

"Many men find this to be quite a challenge, but the reward is that it does bring excellent results. Before long, the lowered vibration of your voice will speed up the vortex in the throat. That, in turn, will help speed up the vortex in the sexual center, which is near the body's doorway to vital life energy. As the upward flow of this energy increases, the throat vortex will speed up still more, helping the voice to go still lower and so on.

"There are young men who appear to be robust and virile now, but who, unfortunately, will not remain that way for long. That is because their voices never fully matured and remained rather high. These individuals, as well as the older ones I've been talking about, can get wonderful results by consciously making the effort to lower their voices. In a younger person, this will help to preserve virility, while in the older one, it will help to renew it.

"Some time ago I came across an excellent voice exercise. Like other effective things, it is quite simple. Whenever you are by yourself or where there is sufficient noise to drown your voice so you won't disturb others, practice saying in a low tone, partly through the nose, 'Mimmm-Mimmm-Mimmm-Mimmm.' Repeat it again and again, lowering your voice in steps, until you've forced it as low as you possibly can. It's effective to do this first thing in the morning when the voice already tends to be in a lower register. Then make an effort to hold your voice in a low pitch for the rest of the day.

"Once you start making progress, practice in the bathroom, so you can hear your voice reverberate. Then try to get the same effect in a larger room. When the vibration of your voice is intensified, it will cause the other vortexes in the body to speed up, especially the second one in the sexual center and the sixth and seventh in the head.

"In older women, the voice can also become high and shrill, and it should be toned down in this same manner. Of course, a woman's voice is naturally higher than a man's, and women should not attempt to lower their voices to the point of sounding masculine. In fact, it would be beneficial for a woman whose voice is abnormally masculine to attempt to raise her voice pitch, using the method already described.

"The lamas chant in unison, sometimes for hours, in a low register. The significance of this is not the chanting itself or the meaning of their words. It is the vibration of their voices and its effect on the seven vortexes.

"Now," said the Colonel after pausing a moment, "everything I've taught you so far has concerned the seven vortexes. But now I'd like to discuss a few things that can make you all much younger, even though they do not directly affect the vortexes.

"If it were possible to suddenly take an aging man or woman out of a decrepit old body and place him or her in a young, new one about twenty-five years of age, I'd be willing to bet that he or she would continue to act old and to hold on to the attitudes that helped bring on old age in the first place.

"Though most people will complain about advancing age, the truth is they get dubious pleasure out of growing old and all the handicaps that come with it. Needless to say, this attitude isn't going to make them any younger. If an older person truly wants to grow younger, they must think, act, and behave like a younger person and eliminate the attitudes and mannerisms of old age.

"The first thing to pay attention to is your posture. Straighten up! When you first started this class, some of you were so bent over that you looked like question marks. But as vitality began returning and your spirits improved, your posture improved also. That was fine, but don't stop now. Think about your posture as you go about your daily activities. Straighten your back, throw your chest out, pull in your chin, and hold your head high. Right away you have eliminated twenty years from your appearance and forty years from your behavior.

"Also, get rid of the mannerisms of old age. When you walk, know first where you are going, then start out and go directly there. Don't shuffle; pick up your feet and stride. Keep one eye on the place where you're going and the other on everything you pass.

"At the Himalayan monastery, there was a man, like myself a Westerner, who acted like a man of twenty-five and didn't look a day over thirty-five years of age. He was actually more than a hundred years old. If I told you how much over a hundred, you wouldn't believe me.

"In order for you to achieve this kind of miracle, you must first desire to do so. Then you must accept the idea that it is not only probable, but absolutely certain that you will. As long as the goal of growing younger is an impossible dream to you, it will remain just that. But once you fully embrace the wonderful reality that you can indeed become younger in appearance, health, and attitude, and once you energize that reality with focused desire, you have already taken your first drink of the healing waters of the fountain of youth.

"The five simple rites which I have taught you are a tool or a device that can enable you to achieve your own personal miracle. After all, it is the simple things of life which are most powerful and effective. If you continue to perform these rites to the best of your ability, you will be ever so richly rewarded.

"It has been most gratifying to see each of you improve from day to day," concluded the Colonel. "I have taught you all that I can for the present. But as the Five Rites continue to do their work, they will open doors to further learning and progress in the future. In the meantime, there are others who need the information which I have taught you, and it is time for me to be on my way to them."

At this the Colonel bade us farewell. This extraordinary man had earned a very special place in our hearts, and so, of course, we were sorry to see him go. But we were also glad to know that before long others would be sharing the priceless information which he had so generously shared with us. We considered ourselves fortunate indeed. For in all of history, few have been privileged to learn the ancient secret of the fountain of youth.

PUBLISHER'S NOTE
THE LOST CHAPTER

The original 1939 edition of this book ended with the conclusion of Part Four. However, eight years later in 1947, the text was revised and expanded with the addition of Part Five, titled *Mantram-Mind Magic*. No copy of the 1947 edition was known to have survived, until one was discovered among the author's personal papers in 1994.

This edition is the first to reinstate the author's 1947 revisions and his elusive Part Five which—to those who knew it had once existed—had become known as "the lost chapter."

PART FIVE

All that is comes from the mind;
it is based on the mind,
it is fashioned by the mind.

—The Pali Canon c. 500–250 B.C.

Now and then the Himalaya Club would receive a short but interesting communication from Colonel Bradford. He was lecturing before groups here and there throughout the world, and he did not stay long in any one place.

One day we received quite a long letter. It contained new information of considerable interest and was intended for all of the club members.

The title of Colonel Bradford's letter, *Mantram-Mind Magic,* aroused some curiosity, since the word *Mantram* was unknown to most members of the group, though some vaguely recalled having seen it somewhere in print. Colonel Bradford's letter explained:

"There is a slight difference between the words *man-*

tra and *mantram*. Both are taken from a Sanskrit word meaning *instrument of thought.* The difference is this: a mantram is a vocalized instrument of thought, while a mantra is silent.

"Whether you realize it or not, you create and shape your life with your thoughts. All things that become part of your physical reality are first created in the mind from the raw material called *thought*. Because it is an *instrument of thought,* a mantram is a tool which you can use to help shape your life as you wish it to be.

"Now, in order to use mantrams to your advantage, you need to first understand the mind and how it works. Nowadays, the term *subconscious mind* is one that's frequently heard but seldom understood. Instead of *subconsciousness,* the lamas use a word that could be translated as *superconsciousness*—consciousness of a higher order. The job of the *superconscious mind* is to take thought, which is pure energy, and give it physical shape in the material world.

"Whole books could be written on the subject, but just now the important thing for you to remember is this: your superconscious mind is a willing and eager servant whom you command by way of your thought patterns. When you think a thought, you issue a command. Your servant obeys by manifesting the thought in the physical world where it becomes the things and events in your life. Thus, physical reality is a mirror of your thought patterns. Change your thought patterns, and you change the reflection in the mirror. In other words, you change your life.

"This concept, as simple as it is, is a stumbling block for many people. They point to some unhappy or even tragic event in their lives and refuse to believe that they could have created it with their own thoughts.

"But if you examine your thoughts closely, you're likely to discover negative patterns competing with positive ones. In one breath you'll say, 'I want to achieve happiness.' But in the next breath you'll give yourself a thousand and one reasons to be unhappy: your job is stressful; the weather is unpleasant; bills are piling up; you're overweight; the neighbors are noisy; you are late for an appointment; and on and on. So while your stated goal is happiness, your thoughts are working overtime to create just the opposite.

"A mantram is something you can use to unify your thought patterns and bring them into alignment with your highest and best desires. To start using this powerful tool, you must first clearly identify the rewards which life is to deliver to your doorstep.

"There's a very simple mental exercise that can help

you accomplish this. It takes only a few minutes, so I suggest that you repeat it every month or so. Sit down and make a written list of the things you desire most. Don't reason as to what you *ought* to want. Instead, jot down your desires quickly, including everything that comes to mind.

"Now examine your list carefully and ask yourself what rewards each of your stated desires must bring you. The rewards are what you're really after, so write them down also. For example, if you wrote, 'I desire a better job,' what you really want are the rewards of a better job. Maybe you want the fulfillment that comes from putting to good use special talents and training you have. Perhaps you want a bigger paycheck and the feeling of security that comes with that. Or maybe you want the pleasure of working in a friendly, relaxed environment.

"The rewards you want should always be expressed in terms of feelings. Feelings, both bitter and sweet, are the fruits of your lifetime experience. They are the prize. When you depart this world, you leave behind your material treasures. But your feelings remain with you always. So choose with care those which you wish to have as lasting companions.

"Now review your list of desires and the rewards you wish to achieve. Read it top to bottom, and as you do, search for just two or three words or phrases to summarize everything. This may seem impossible at first. But once you look closely, you'll see groups of seemingly different desires and rewards all aimed at a common goal. Separate your desires into two or three such groups and find a word or phrase to capsulize each one. To use a simple example, if you desire a better house, an expensive automobile, and a new wardrobe, the fundamental goal behind all three is *abundance* or *prosperity*.

"By now you should have a clear picture of your fundamental goals, so put them all together and state them in a brief command. Make the command positive, short, and to the point. For example, 'I demand happiness, power, and prosperity right now.' And there you have it. When your command is spoken aloud, it becomes a mantram, or plainly stated, a device you can use to stimulate your superconscious mind into action.

"The word *power* is a good one, because it will help bring about health, strength, and vitality in your physical body. And on a mental level, it will empower you to become master of your own destiny. *Right now* at the end of your command tells your superconscious mind when you want things to happen: *NOW*. It tells your superconscious mind to get busy immediately manifesting your desires.

"Now that you have a mantram, putting it to use is as simple as can be. All you need to do is speak it aloud with conviction. Don't be timid. Feel the power of your voice and speak as if you are commanding a magic genie who will bring you whatever you desire. Once you have spoken your mantram aloud with unwavering conviction and resolve, you've done all that's needed.

"Speak your mantram just before going to sleep at night and upon waking in the morning. Then form the habit of repeating it at regular intervals throughout the day. If you find yourself in front of a mirror, gaze directly into the reflection of your own eyes and repeat your mantram with firm confidence.

"Then, as you go about your daily life, pay close attention to all the things you think and say. Be alert for negative thoughts or words that will send conflicting commands to your superconscious mind. They will undo the positive force of your mantram, so when you detect them, stop, take a deep breath, and cancel the negative thoughts or words by speaking your mantram with steadfast resolve.

"Of course, if you are in the presence of other people, you can't all of a sudden blurt out, 'I desire happiness, power, and prosperity right now!' In such a case, I would suggest that you use a mantra. All that's needed is to repeat your mantra inwardly and contemplate the meaning of the words. Since it isn't reinforced by the power of the voice, a mantra isn't quite as effective as a spoken Mantram, but it will get splendid results nevertheless.

"Whether you're using a mantram or a mantra, an important thing to remember is this: when you command the superconscious mind, you must focus only on the end result which you desire. Never try to dictate *how* superconsciousness will accomplish its miracles.

"The superconscious mind is far more clever and resourceful than you can possibly imagine. If it is headed off in one direction, it is not discouraged and does not give up, for it knows that there are ten thousand other ways to achieve a desired goal. If, through your own thoughts and preconceptions, you try to tell the superconscious mind how to do its work, you will only limit its options and restrict the magic which can unfold.

"The superconscious realm of your mind is a magnificent thing. It takes great delight in working to accomplish literally anything you desire. Desire is a very strong force, and when you use it to stimulate the superconscious mind into action, it will be thrilled to bring you your heart's desire in ways you never dreamed possible.

"Another thing you should know is this: the superconscious realm of the mind does not judge your thoughts before it responds to them. It does not differentiate between pain or pleasure, sorrow or happiness, grief or joy. A better way to state it is, no feelings or emotions are pleasant or unpleasant to the superconscious mind. Its job is to transform thought patterns into matter—*all thought patterns*. And it could not possibly do the job it is meant to do if it were to first judge your thoughts good or bad, happy or unhappy, worthy or unworthy.

"In short, the wonderfully simple secret which can help everybody achieve whatever they desire is this: change your thought patterns, and you change your life. If you think thrilling thoughts, the superconscious mind will flood your life with thrilling things, instead of the miserable things in life.

"Now, the superconscious mind is an extraordinary thing, but it cannot make use of meaningless thoughts. So, to be effective your mantram must speak clearly to you in a personal and meaningful way. To make sure that it does, there are two things which you should keep in mind:

"First, as you grow and evolve, it's important for your mantram to do the same. So whenever you feel that your personal growth has led to changes in your goals and objectives, revise your Mantram to reflect these changes.

"Second, your Mantram must be spoken in a language which is *completely familiar to you*. I mention this because certain teachers from the East advocate Mantrams which are very well and good for people who speak the language of the East. But they are useless to people who do not understand them. Even if you are told the meaning of the words, they are just so much gibberish to your superconscious mind, and as a result no good will be accomplished.

"There is one exception, however. One particular word which comes from the East has a magical effect upon the superconscious mind and also upon the brain and the central nervous system. The word is *OM*. Actually, it's not so much a word as a sound, for its value is in its tonal vibration, not in its meaning. Thus, anyone using OM for vibratory purposes will receive a special benefit, no matter what language they speak or understand—anyone, that is, who is ready for vibrations that are high and powerful.

"The use of OM—I shall call it Rite Number Seven—can produce exceptional results in the right individual. When it is intoned correctly, its vibratory frequency has a very powerful stimulating effect on the pineal gland, which is related to the seventh and highest vortex. However, your pineal gland should not be stimulated into great action unless the life you are leading is focused on a higher plane. Just as a seed cannot sprout in barren ground, vibrations of a higher order cannot flourish in a consciousness that is not yet ready to receive them. Do not attempt to practice Rite Number Seven until the first five rites have helped elevate and attune your physical and mental being. Your vibration must be sufficiently high, so that you are beyond the use of all habit-forming drugs, including alcohol and nicotine in any and all forms.

"To prepare yourself, watch your diet. It should be low in fats, and you should avoid sweetenings of all kinds, since they contain sugar which is a first cousin to alcohol. Starches can also be detrimental, unless they are thoroughly masticated. But once they are predigested in the mouth, starches are not harmful if taken in sensible quantities.

"And it's especially important to increase the amount of water you consume. The average healthy person should drink about three quarts of pure water (twelve eight-ounce glasses) daily. If you are larger or smaller than average, drink more or less. However, do not begin drinking so much water all at once. Instead, increase your water intake very gradually over a period of sixty days. Water not only helps to cleanse your body of wastes and impurities, it is also a splendid conductor of electrical current and sound vibration. Your increased use of water should take place first and for at least one month. Then you can begin to practice Rite Number Seven with good results.

"To practice this rite, stand on the floor or sit in a comfortable armchair. Relax completely, but do not slouch down. Keep your posture erect and hold your chin up, so that your vocal cords are not restricted in any way. You can even lie flat on your back on a firm bed or on the floor, if you wish, but do not prop a pillow under your head. That would thrust the head forward and cramp the vocal cords.

"OM is pronounced like the word *home,* but without the *h.* To intone this magical sound correctly, begin by taking a very deep breath, but don't fill your lungs so much that they are bursting with air. Then, using a good, deep, full-bodied voice, sound the vowel 'Oh-h-h . . .' Your jaw should be halfway open; your lips should be in a rounded position; and your tongue should be retracted and low in the mouth, but elevated toward the rear of the mouth. Sustain the 'Oh-h-h . . .' sound for about five seconds. Then continue sounding your voice as you close and relax your jaw, close and flatten your lips, and relax the tongue in a flat position, forming the sound 'M-m-m-m-m-m . . .' Sustain this sound for about ten seconds.

"When you sound 'Oh-h-h . . . ,' you should feel your voice resonate through the chest cavities. When you sound 'M-m-m-m-m-m . . . ,' you should feel it resonate through the nasal cavities. When done correctly, the two will blend together in one continuous 'O-h-h-M-m-m-m-m-m . . .' sound.

"When you are finished, relax and take one or two deep breaths before repeating OM. Three or four times in succession is quite sufficient. Do not overdo a good thing. And stop if you begin to feel the least bit light-headed or dizzy. After an hour or so, perform the OMs again several times. When you are new to this rite, do not perform it more than ten times in one day, even if you experience no light-headedness. Too much pineal stimulation for a beginner is not a positive thing.

"It is best if you do not speak your mantram and perform Rite Number Seven in the same session. Rite Number Seven should be performed only when the mind is quiet and free of thoughts. However, you can combine Rite Number Seven with a mantra to excellent advantage. When you are sounding the 'Oh-h-h . . .' part of OM for five seconds, allow your mind to be thoroughly still and quiet. Then, as you intone 'M-m-m-m-m-m . . .' for ten seconds, repeat your mantra mentally several times.

"The mantra should be prepared before you begin, and it may be the same as your mantram. Be sure that it is stated in the form of a command calling for the fulfillment of your fundamental goals. And be absolutely certain that it does not contain any negative thoughts or words that will cancel the good of your efforts.

"Because this rite is so powerful, it is intended for mature individuals only. It most certainly should not be used by anyone under the age of twenty-one. And it will be most helpful to those who have reached the season of life when wisdom begins to ripen.

"In fact, once they start the job of increasing their vibrations, older men and women often make better progress than younger ones, partly because they have learned to see beyond the distractions and illusions of the material world where joys are as fleeting as dry leaves in the wind. They know that life's true rewards are to be found not outside themselves, but in the world that lies within.

"On their inward journeys, the Illuminati—the wise men of old—have all used Rite Number Seven to raise the vibration of their minds and of their physical bodies as well. When you do the same, you will move forward to achieve youth of mind and youth of body, together with the treasure of wisdom.

"In closing, I encourage you to take up the challenge and begin anew right where you are. For though you have made splendid progress and though your accomplishments are many, the rewards you have earned are nothing compared to those that await you once you begin your inward journey. When you do, you will not turn back, for great things lie just ahead, well within your grasp.

Faithfully yours, Colonel Bradford"

After receiving this letter, the members of the Himalaya Club never again heard from Colonel Bradford. His whereabouts were unknown and my best efforts to locate him proved unsuccessful. The only thing that can be said with certainty is that the Colonel's travels took him to places unknown, to adventures untold, and to marvels which one can only imagine.

PUBLISHER'S
AFTERWORD

Just ten years after Peter Kelder's book first appeared, China invaded Tibet and claimed it as part of the Chinese "motherland." In the decade that followed, it laid waste to the small mountain kingdom, devastating a culture which had been thousands of years in the making.

Inflamed by the Cultural Revolution, the Chinese began systematically destroying Tibetan Buddhism across the land. Monasteries were ruined. Monks and lamas were murdered. Many ancient monasteries were literally blown up by dynamite or mortar shell. The roofs of hermitages were removed, so that they would be quickly destroyed by the elements. Invaluable spiritual texts were burned or used as toilet paper. Libraries were ransacked. Religious objects were turned into rubble. Once-venerated temples were used as pigsties and slaughterhouses. Sacred clay images were stamped into dust or made into building bricks. Of the approximately 600,000 monks living in Tibet before the Chinese invasion, only an estimated 7,000 survived; as many as 100,000 fled the country. Within three years of the Chinese invasion, Tibet was scarred by ruins, resembling the bombed cities of Europe after World War II.

Perhaps even worse, China introduced an estimated seven million Han Chinese into Tibet, making native Tibetans a minority in their own country.

Some characterize this desecration of Tibet as the Buddhist Holocaust. Since the invasion of Tibet, an estimated 1.2 million Tibetans have died, victims of violence, execution, imprisonment, torture, starvation, and suicide. Thousands more have fled Tibet. They struggle to survive in refugee settlements under conditions of extreme poverty and deprivation.

TIBET AND TIBETAN BUDDHISM TODAY

Today, hundreds of Tibetans are being held as political prisoners in one of Lhasa's four jails. The situation now resembles the mood of Eastern Europe during the Communist era. There are numerous Chinese spies and informers in Tibet, free speech is almost nonexistent, and many Tibetans live in fear and desperation. As the year 2000 approaches, Tibet is the world's longest-occupied (and largest) sovereign state.

For many in the West, Tibet's spiritual and political leader, Tenzin Gyatso, the Fourteenth Dalai Lama, is the face of that shattered and struggling nation. In 1959, he was persuaded to flee to Dharamsala, India, where he established and still maintains a government-in-exile. In spite of the atrocities committed by the Chinese, he believes that the cultivation of compassion and nonviolent diplomacy is the only route to world peace and the only path for the Tibetan people. The recipient of the 1989 Nobel Peace Prize, he recently told a reporter for *The New York Times* that "the Tibetan resistance has worldwide support because it is nonviolent." He also said that he is hopeful for the eventual restitution of the Tibetan homeland. In his autobiography, he wrote: "Thus, despite the continuing tragedy of Tibet, I find much good in the world."

There are a number of organizations dedicated to advancing the Tibetan cause. To learn how you can help, please contact the following:

TIBET HOUSE
22 West 15th Street
New York, NY 10111
Tel: 212-213-5592
Fax: 212-213-6408

Tibet House is devoted to efforts to save Tibetan culture from the threat of extinction. The Tibet House

Cultural Center in midtown Manhattan hosts exhibits and cultural events, and its Tibetan Studies Program offers classes in Tibetan language, art, history, medicine, and spiritual sciences. Tibet House also maintains an archive of old Tibetan photographs and a program to conserve art and artifacts.

THE TIBET FUND
241 East 32 Street
New York, NY 10016
Tel: 212-213-5011
Fax: 212-779-9245

The Tibet Fund addresses the needs of the Tibetan refugee community in India, Nepal, and elsewhere. The Tibet Fund's primary mission is to help support and strengthen this community through programs in education, health, economic and community development, and religion. A donor may sponsor a monk or nun at a monastic institution or a child at a refugee school.

TIBETAN RIGHTS CAMPAIGN
P.O. Box 31966
Seattle, WA 98103–0066

Tel: 206-547-1015

Fax: 206-547-3758

The Tibetan Rights Campaign (TRC) works to raise awareness of the plight of the Tibetan people and to advance their struggle for human rights, democracy, and independence. Their work includes cultural events; talks, videos, and slide shows; *Tibet Monitor,* a monthly news report on developments concerning Tibet; a lending library of books on Tibet; and quarterly membership meetings.

INTERNATIONAL CAMPAIGN FOR
TIBET
1825 K Street NW, Ste. 520
Washington, DC 20006
Tel: 202-785-1515
Fax: 202-785-4343

The International Campaign for Tibet (ICT) is a nonpartisan, public interest group dedicated to promoting human rights and democratic freedoms for the people of Tibet. ICT believes that governments and people around the world need accurate information on current conditions in Tibet.

A P P E N D I X

Any new exercise program should be undertaken with care. Consult a qualified medical practitioner before attempting the exercises described in this book.

Jeff Migdow, M.D., who has had extensive practical experience with the Five Rites, offers the following precautionary advice. However, his list of precautions is by no means comprehensive, and it should not be viewed as a substitute for advice from your own personal physician.

RITE NUMBER ONE Spinning can cause nausea, headache, and a loss of balance. Initially, when you first begin doing this rite, spin slowly. Always go clockwise.

Because spinning might aggravate the following conditions, seek professional advice if you have multiple sclerosis, Parkinson's or a Parkinson-like disease, Ménière's disease, vertigo, seizure disorders, pregnancy with nausea, or are taking drugs that can cause dizziness. If you have an enlarged heart, a heart valve problem, or have suffered a heart attack within the past three months, do not attempt this rite without your doctor's explicit permission.

RITE NUMBER TWO If you have ulcers, lower back pain, neck pain, high blood pressure that is being controlled with medication, weak abdominal muscles, excessive tension or stiffness in shoulders or legs, multiple sclerosis, Parkinson's or a Parkinson-like disease, fibromyositis, or chronic fatigue syndrome, do this rite very slowly and increase the number of repetitions by one or two per week. Menstruating women should be aware that it may aggravate cramping and interrupt or stop menstrual flow.

If you have hiatal hernia, hernia, hyperthyroid condition, Ménière's disease, vertigo, or a seizure disorder, ask your health care practitioner whether this exercise is safe for you. It may be contraindicated if you are pregnant, have had abdominal surgery within six months, or if you have uncontrolled high blood pressure or hyperthyroidism, severe arthritis of the spine, or disc disease; get your doctor's permission first. If you have an enlarged heart, heart valve problems, or have suffered a heart attack within the past three months, do not do this rite without your doctor's explicit approval.

RITE NUMBER THREE If you are taking medication for high blood pressure, you should not allow the head to be positioned lower than the heart.

If you have lower back or neck pain, weak abdominal muscles, recurring headaches, multiple sclerosis, Parkinson's or a Parkinson-like disease, fibromyositis, or chronic fatigue syndrome, you should perform each repetition of this movement very slowly and add only one or two repetitions per week.

If you suffer from hernia, hiatal hernia, uncontrolled high blood pressure, severe arthritis of the spine, disc disease, hyperthyroidism, Ménière's disease, vertigo, or seizure disorders, check with your health care practitioner about whether this rite is safe for you to do. Pregnant women and those who have had abdominal surgery within six months should seek advice from a doctor. If you have an enlarged heart, a heart valve problem, or have suffered a heart attack within the last three months, do not do this rite without your doctor's explicit approval.

RITE NUMBER FOUR Do this rite slowly and add only one or two repetitions per week if you have high blood pressure that is being controlled with medication, ulcers, lower back pain, neck pain, weak abdominal muscles, weakness or stiffness in the shoulders or legs, multiple sclerosis, Parkinson's or a Parkinson-like disease, fibromyositis, carpal tunnel syndrome, or chronic fatigue syndrome. It may aggravate cramping or stop menstrual flow if done during menses.

If you are diagnosed with any of the following conditions, this rite should be done with the approval of your health care practitioner: hernia, hiatal hernia, hyperthyroidism, Ménière's disease, vertigo, and seizure disorders. It may be contraindicated if you are pregnant, have had abdominal surgery within six months, suffer from severe hernias or hiatal hernias, uncontrolled high blood pressure, severe arthritis of the spine, disc disease; seek your doctor's advice before trying to do this rite. If you have an enlarged heart, a heart valve problem, or have suffered a heart attack within the past three months, do not do this rite without your doctor's explicit approval.

RITE NUMBER FIVE Do this movement slowly and add only one or two repetitions per week if you have ulcers, lower back pain, neck pain, weak abdominal muscles, shoulder or leg stiffness or weakness, multiple sclerosis, Parkinson's or a Parkinson-like disease, fibromyositis, carpal tunnel syndrome, or chronic fatigue syndrome.

Seek an informed medical opinion before doing this rite if you have high blood pressure, hiatal hernia, hernia, severe arthritis of the spine, disc disease, hyperthyroidism, Ménière's disease, vertigo, or a seizure disorder. It may be contraindicated during pregnancy, if you've had abdominal surgery within six months, if medication is not effectively controlling your blood pressure, or if you have severe hernia. If you have an enlarged heart, a heart valve problem, or have suffered a heart attack within the past three months, do not do this rite without your doctor's explicit approval.

GENERAL ADVICE Performing the Five Rites can set many physical changes in motion. Initially, the rites, which stimulate circulation, can have a dramatic detoxifying effect, and that's one reason for gradually working into the full routine of twenty-one repetitions. Once you begin, you may notice that your urine is a darker color or has a strong odor. It may sting or burn when you urinate. Women might develop a vaginal infection. You may notice an unpleasant change in the smell of your sweat or a slight rash on the skin. You might develop a slight upper respiratory infection or discomfort in your joints. These symptoms occur as the body begins to excrete poisons and pollutants which have been deposited in organs, joints, and mucous membranes. Although they are temporary and should be viewed as normal, check with your doctor to be sure these symptoms do not require medical attention.

Jeff Migdow, M.D., is on the staff of the Kripalu Center in Lenox, Massachusetts, one of the largest yoga-oriented health care facilities in the world. His comments are excerpted from Ancient Secret of the Fountain of Youth, Book 2—*a companion to the book you are now reading, which will be published by Doubleday in 1999. In it, Dr. Migdow contributes a chapter titled "The Five Rites and Yoga: Exercises for Renewed Health and Longevity."*

EXPERTS SHOW YOU THE WAY TO RAPID PROGRESS:

The Five Rites on Video

Now, your own personal instructor can help you get maximum benefit from the Five Tibetan Rites in the comfort and convenience of your own home.

In *Ancient Secret of the Fountain of Youth, THE VIDEO,* yoga and fitness experts Bija Bennett and Rory Reich lead you step-by-step through each exercise, giving you a wealth of tips and techniques for fast and lasting progress.

- Learn to start with modified exercises that will have you doing all the Five Rites from the first day.
- Fine-tune your technique for rapid advancement.
- Find out how to avoid problems and mistakes that limit your progress.
- Discover hidden health benefits in each of the Rites.

Visually stunning and beautifully produced, *Ancient Secret of the Fountain of Youth, THE VIDEO,* features music by internationally acclaimed Tibetan recording artist Nawang Khechog.

For an experience that's not to be missed, order your copy of *Ancient Secret of the Fountain of Youth, THE VIDEO,* now.

Just $19.95 plus shipping★
Available in stores, or for fastest service
CALL TOLL-FREE 888–855–5400.

To order by mail: Send a check or money order for $23.95 (includes Priority Shipping) to:

THE VIDEO
P.O. Box 2299
Gig Harbor, WA 98335

(Washington State residents please pay $25.96, which includes state sales tax.)

★Price subject to change without notice.